Preface

MCQs (Ear, Nose, Throat and Head and Neck Surgery) for Undergraduate Medical Students has two main roles. First, we aim to provide a bank of questions for examination practice, as familiarity breeds confidence.

Second, we want to provide an informative text with taking advantage of the collective knowledge from our colleagues in the Ear, Nose and Throat and Head and Neck Surgery specialty.

We sincerely hope that this book helps you in the build-up to your examination and wish you all the best in your future medical career.

A. K. Soe and Mehdee Hassan

1. Peritonsillar abscess is also known as
    (A) Retropharyngeal abscess
    (B) Tonsillar abscess
    (C) Quinsy
    (D) Ludwig's angina
    (E) Thornwaldt's abscess

2. Cranial accessory nerve supplies
    (A) Palate
    (B) Pharynx
    (C) Palatoglossus
    (D) Sternocleidomastoid
    (E) Tongue

3. All muscles of tongue are supplied by hypoglossal nerve
    except
    (A) Myoglossus
    (B) Palatoglossus
    (C) Genioglossus
    (D) Hyoglossus
    (E) Styloglossus

4. Which implant is used in nasopharyngeal carcinoma?
    (A) Caesium
    (B) I-131
    (C) Gold
    (D) Iridium
    (E) All

5. A gentleman aged 60 years old has foul breath, he
    regurgitates food that is eaten 3 days ago. Likely diagnosis is
    (A) Zenker's diverticulum
    (B) Meckel's diverticulum
    (C) Scleroderma
    (D) Achalasia cardia
    (E) Laryngocele

6. During inspiration the main current of airflow in a normal nasal cavity is through
   (A) Middle part of the cavity in middle meatus in a parabolic curve
   (B) Lower part of the cavity in the inferior meatus in a parabolic curve
   (C) Superior part of the cavity in the superior meatus
   (D) Through olfactory area
   (E) Inferior part of the cavity in the inferior meatus

7. Which is not a synonym of inverted papilloma
   (A) Ringertz tumor
   (B) Epithelial cell papilloma
   (C) Transitional cell papilloma
   (D) Schneiderian papilloma
   (E) Columnar cell papilloma

8. Which of these is not an indication for use of nasal steroid sprays
   (A) Allergic fungal sinusitis
   (B) Acute fungal sinusitis
   (C) Non allergic vasomotor rhinitis
   (D) Anosmia
   (E) Allergic rhinitis

9. The incidence of choanal atresia is
   (A) One per 1000 live birth
   (B) One per 4000 live birth
   (C) One per 7000 live birth
   (D) One per 200 live birth
   (E) One per 10000 live birth

10. Adenoidectomy should be avoided in
    (A) Sub mucous cleft palate
    (B) Bifid uvula
    (C) Significant history of nasal regurgitation as an infant
    (D) All of the above

(E) None of the above

11. Sinus which is not present at birth is
    (A) Maxillary sinus
    (B) Frontal sinus
    (C) Ethmoid sinus
    (D) Sphenoid sinus

12. Nasal perforation in bony part is caused by
    (A) Atrophic rhinitis
    (B) Systemic lupus erythromatosis
    (C) Tuberculosis
    (D) Cocaine abuse
    (E) Syphilis

13. Artery of epistaxis is the name given to
    (A) Sphenopalatine artery
    (B) Superior labial artery
    (C) Anterior ethmoidal artery
    (D) Posterior ethmoidal artery
    (E) Greater palatine artery

14. Direction of nasolacrimal duct is
    (A) Downward forward and medially
    (B) Downward backward and medially
    (C) Downward forward and laterally
    (D) Downward backward and laterally

15. True regarding rhinosporidiosis
    (A) Seen only in immunocompromised patients
    (B) Most common organism is Klebsiella Rhinoscleromatis
    (C) Present as nasal polyps
    (D) Can be diagnosed by isolation of organism

16. Taste sensation of posterior one third of tongue is innervated by
    (A) Lingual nerve

(B) Chorda tympani nerve

(C) Glosopharyngeal nerve

(D) Vagus nerve

(E) Hypoglossal nerve

17. Oroantral fistula is caused by following, except
    (A) CA maxilla
    (B) Caldwell Luc operation
    (C) Dental extraction
    (D) Maxillectomy

18. Ethmoid polyp is characterized by the followings, except
    (A) Viral in origin
    (B) Multiple
    (C) Antihistamine is effective
    (D) Surgery is treatment of choice

19. What is the embryological etiology of choanal atresia
    (A) Persistence of buccopharyngeal membrane
    (B) Failure of involution of buccopharyngeal membrane
    (C) Persistence of epithelial cells which proliferate within the nasal cavities during sixth to eight week of intrauterine life
    (D) All the statements are true
    (E) None of the statements are true

20. Which of these is characteristic of choanal atresia
    (A) Disappearance of cyanosis when the child cries, in a cyanosed child at rest
    (B) Appearance of cyanosis when the child cries, in a normal child at rest
    (C) Cyanosed child irrespective of crying, but colour improves during sleep
    (D) All the statements are true
    (E) None of the statements are true

21. Changes seen in cell morphology of nasal epithelium in a case of choanal atresia
    (A) Uneven thickening of mucosal surface
    (B) Thickening of basal membrane
    (C) Presence of ciliary abnormalities including compound cilia, cilia excessive cytoplasm and ciliary structures with loss of peripheral membrane
    (D) All the statements are true
    (E) None of the statements are true

22. What is the CT scan finding in a case of choanal atresia
    (A) Thicken vomer
    (B) Bowing of lateral wall of nasal cavity
    (C) Fusion of bony elements in the region of choanal
    (D) All the above statements
    (E) None of the above statements

23. Which of these anomalies is not related with choanal atresia
    (A) Cardiac valvular defects
    (B) Mental retardation
    (C) Renal agenesis
    (D) Genital hypoplasia in male
    (E) Ear deformities including deafness

24. Choanal atresia is
    (A) A common pediatric embryological anomaly
    (B) A neonatal emergency
    (C) Uncurable embryological anomaly with significant after effects
    (D) All the statements are correct
    (E) None of the statements are true

25. The diagnosis of choanal atresia is confirmed by
    (A) Failure to pass catheter through the nose to oropharynx on either side
    (B) Present or absence of blast/bubbles in either nares

(C) Ct scan findings of bony or membranous plate in region of choanal
(D) All the statements are true
(E) None of the statements is true

26. Emergency management of choanal atresia is
    (A) Insertion of standard neonatal water's airway into infant's mouth between teeth
    (B) Feeding through indwelling nasogastric tube
    (C) Tracheostomy
    (D) All the statements are emergency management
    (E) None of these statements is true

27. Which of these is used as management modality for choanal atresia
    (A) Endoscopic resection
    (B) Mitomycin C
    (C) Stents
    (D) All the statements are true
    (E) None of the statements is true

28. Commonest cause of acute sinusitis
    (A) Swimming and diving
    (B) Acute rhinitis
    (C) Dental infection
    (D) Nasal tumor

29. Alkaline nasal douche contains all excepts
    (A) Sodium bicarbonate
    (B) Sodium biborate
    (C) Sodium chloride
    (D) Glucose

30. Caldwell view can visualize
    (A) Sphenoid sinus
    (B) Maxillary sinus
    (C) Ethmoid and frontal sinus

(D) Nasal bones

31. Which of these statements describes Schuller's view best
    (A) Cephalo caudal beam makes an angle of 30 degrees to the saggital
    (B) 15 degrees cephalo caudal beam
    (C) View is taken such that long axis of petrous bone lies parallel to the film
    (D) Antero posterior view with 30 degrees tilt from above and in front

32. Which of these can be used for Water's view
    (A) Occipito frontal view
    (B) Occipito mental view
    (C) Submental vertical view
    (D) 30 degrees cephalo caudal to saggital view

33. Trans orbital view is useful for study of
    (A) Coalescent mastoiditis
    (B) Congenital bilateral sclerotic mastoids
    (C) Temporal bone malignancies
    (D) Acoustic neuroma

34. Stenver's view is useful for the study of which of the following structures
    (A) External auditory canal
    (B) Middle ear
    (C) Cochlea
    (D) Mastoid antrum
    (E) Petrous apex

35. Which of these arteries is not a part of Kiesselbach's plexus
    (A) Superior labial artery
    (B) Greater palatine artery
    (C) Sphenopalatine artery
    (D) Anterior ethmoidal artery
    (E) Posterior ethmoidal artery

36. Which of these arteries which constitute Little's area is not a branch of external carotid artery
    (A) Superior labial artery
    (B) Greater palatine artery
    (C) Sphenopalatine artery
    (D) Anterior ethmoidal artery

37. Location of Woodruff's area
    (A) Posterior end of middle turbinate
    (B) Posterior end of inferior turbinate
    (C) Anterior end of middle turbinate
    (D) Anterior part of nasal septum

38. Which of these is more likely to cause sudden spontaneous onset profuse epistaxis
    (A) Finger nail trauma
    (B) Atrophic rhinitis
    (C) Maggots in the nasal cavity
    (D) Juvenile nasopharyngeal carcinoma

39. What is "Trotter's method of management of epistaxis
    (A) Pinching of nose for 5-10 minutes
    (B) Patient made to sit, leaning a little forward over a basin to spit any blood, and breath quietly from mouth
    (C) Cauterization of bleeding vessels with silver nitrate
    (D) Anterior nasal packing

40. Which of these will cause posterior epistaxis
    (A) Finger nail trauma
    (B) Acute bacterial sinusitis
    (C) Syphilis septal perforation
    (D) Uncontrolled hypertension

41. Posterior epistaxis can be managed by which of the following methods
    (A) Posterior nasal packing

(B) Endoscopic cauterization
(C) Epistaxis catheter balloon
(D) All of the above

42. Which of these arteries should be ligated in uncontrolled posterior epistaxis
    (A) External carotid artery
    (B) Maxillary artery
    (C) Anterior ethmoid artery
    (D) Interior carotid artery

43. Which of these statements is not true for management of epistaxis
    (A) No antibiotics need to be prescribed
    (B) In case of anterior nasal packing, prophylactic antibiotics should be given
    (C) Anterior nasal pack can be kept in situ up to 7 days without changing
    (D) Foley's catheter can be used for posterior nasal packing.

44. As part of initial first aid of epistaxis, it is advised to pinch nose. How long should ideally nose be pinched
    (A) 2 minutes
    (B) 2 minutes pinch followed by relaxation of 2 minutes, and continue alternatively
    (C) 5-8 minutes
    (D) 30- 60 minutes

45. Which of the following statements is false in relation to "foreign body in nose in a child"
    (A) Unilateral foul smelling nasal discharge
    (B) Has spontaneous onset profuse epistaxis
    (C) Inanimate is common than animate foreign body
    (D) Instrument preferred for removal of foreign body nose is a Eustachian tube catheter.

46. Gold standard test for diagnosis of CSF rhinorrhea is

(A) Beta 2 microglobulin
(B) Beta 2 transferrin
(C) Thyroglobulin
(D) Transthyretin

47. Which of the following statements is true regarding juvenile nasopharyngeal carcinoma
    (A) Holman Miller sign can be positive
    (B) Surgery is the treatment of choice
    (C) Seen in males
    (D) All the statements are true
    (E) All the statements are false

48. Which of the following is not a part of oral cavity
    (A) Buccal mucosa
    (B) Soft palate
    (C) Gingivobuccal sulcus
    (D) Hard palate

49. An 8 year old child has aspirated foreign body into the trachea. The best initial management is
    (A) Heimlich manoeuvre
    (B) Tracheostomy
    (C) Intubation
    (D) Oxygen with IPPV

50. Which of these best describes "Acute Rhinosinusitis" based on duration of symptoms
    (A) < 7 days
    (B) < 14 days
    (C) 7 days to < = 4 weeks
    (D) < = 4 weeks
    (E) 4 weeks to <= 12 weeks

51. Which of these doesn't form a standard part of classification of rhinosinusitis
    (A) Acute rhinosinusitis

(B) Subacute rhinosinusitis
(C) Chronic rhinosinusitis
(D) Recurrent acute sinusitis
(E) All are standard classifications
52. Which of these is not a major symptom for chronic rhinosinusitis definition
(A) Nasal obstruction
(B) Headache
(C) Facial congestion / fullness
(D) Hyposmia / anosmia
(E) Facial pain / pressure

53. The most common bacteria leading to acute rhinosinusitis
(A) Streptococcus pneumoniae
(B) Hemophilus influenzae
(C) Moraxella catarrhalis
(D) Staphylococcus species

54. Most common bacteria leading to chronic rhinosinusitis
(A) Streptococcus pneumoniae
(B) Hemophilus influenzae
(C) Moraxella catarrhalis
(D) Staphylococcus species

55. Which of the following anatomic variants has been most closely linked with development of chronic rhinosinusitis
(A) Concha bullosa
(B) Nasal septal deflection
(C) Agar nasi cells
(D) Bifid middle turbinate

56. In modified Lund scoring system on CT for sinusitis, which of these cannot be given a score of " 1 "
(A) Frontal sinus
(B) Posterior ethmoid sinus

(C) Osteomeatal complex

(D) Maxillary sinus

57. "Guafenesin" has been suggested to have a role in treatment of chronic rhinosinusitis by some researches. What is the mechanism?

(A) Anti-allergic

(B) Mast cell stabilizer

(C) Mucolytic

(D) Leukotriene receptor antagonist

58. Which of these is the mechanism of action of macrolides in treatment of chronic rhinosinusitis

(A) Gram positive antibiotic effect

(B) Anti-inflammatory effect

(C) Immunomodulator effect

(D) All of the above

59. Gastro esophageal reflux disease as a possible etiology of development of chronic rhinosinusitis is more important in which age group

(A) Pediatric

(B) Adults

(C) Geriatric

(D) GERD cannot cause sinusitis

60. A 3 year old child has been brought with facial lacerations. On examination, he gas some cuts over his right cheek and under the eye. The GCS on initial evaluation is 15. What is the appropriate next investigation?

(A) Skull X rays

(B) Facial X rays

(C) CT scan

(D) MRI

(E) Observation

61. A 22 year old lady has been unwell for some time. She came to the hospital with complaints of fever and painful vesicles in her left ear. What is the most probable diagnosis?
(A) Acne
(B) Herpes zoster
(C) Chicken pox
(D) Insect bite
(E) Cellulitis

62. A 5 year old girl had earache and some yellowish foul smelling discharge, attic perforation and conductive hearing loss. She has no past history of any ear infection. What is the most appropriate diagnosis?
(A) Acute otitis media
(B) Otitis media with effusion
(C) Acquired cholesteatoma
(D) Congenital cholesteatoma
(E) Otitis externa

63. A 10 year old girl presents with hoarseness of the voice. She is a known case of bronchial asthma and has been on oral steroids for a while. What is the most likely cause of hoarseness?
(A) Laryngeal candidiasis
(B) Infective tonsillitis
(C) Laryngeal edema
(D) Allergic drug reaction
(E) Ludwig's angina

64. A young man is brought to the emergency department after a RTA. His GCS on initial evaluation is 6. What is the most appropriate next step?
(A) CT
(B) MRI
(C) IV fluids
(D) Skull X rays
(E) Secure airway

65. A 30 year old man complaints of hoarseness of voice. Examination shows unilateral immobile vocal cord. What is the most probable diagnosis?
(A) Grave disease
(B) Hematoma
(C) Unilateral recurrent laryngeal nerve injury
(D) External laryngeal nerve injury
(E) Tracheomalacia

66. A 44 patient has sudden onset of breathlessness and stridor few minutes after extubation for thyroidectomy. The patient had longstanding goiter for which he underwent the thyroid surgery. What is the most likely diagnosis?
(A) Thyroid storm
(B) Hematoma
(C) Unilateral recurrent laryngeal nerve injury
(D) External laryngeal nerve injury
(E) Tracheomalacia

67. A 20 year old pop star singer complaints of inability to raise the pitch of her voice. She attributes this to the thyroid surgery she underwent a few months back. What is the most likely diagnosis?
(A) Thyroid storm
(B) Bilateral recurrent laryngeal nerve injury
(C) Unilateral recurrent laryngeal nerve injury
(D) External laryngeal nerve injury
(E) Thyroid cyst

68. A child is brought in with high grade fever, runny nose and bark-like cough. He is also drooling. What is the most appropriate next step for this child?
(A) Corticosteroids
(B) Paracetamol
(C) Adrenaline nebulizer
(D) IV antibiotics

(E) Intubation under GA

69. A man presents with muffled hearing and feeling of pressure in ear with tinnitus and vertigo. He also complains of double vision when looking to the right. What is the most appropriate diagnosis?
(A) Meniere's disease
(B) Acoustic neuroma
(C) Acute labyrinthitis
(D) Meningioma
(E) Otosclerosis

70. An old 72 year old lady staying at a nursing home for a few years, with a known hypertension on regular treatment presented with sudden dysphagia while eating with drooling of saliva and regular urgent investigation. What would be your next step?
(A) Barium swallow
(B) Chest CT
(C) Endoscopy
(D) Laryngoscopy
(E) CXR

71. A 32 year old man presents with hearing loss. He also complaints of tinnitus, vertigo and numbness on same half of his face. After Rinne test, air conduction is better than bone conduction. What is the most appropriate investigation for his condition?
(A) Audiometry
(B) CT
(C) MRI
(D) Tympanometry
(E) Weber's test

72. A 31 year old man has bleeding from the nose 10 days following nasal polypectomy. What is the most likely diagnosis?

(A) Nasal infection
(B) Coagulation disorder
(C) Allergic rhinitis
(D) Sinusitis
(E) Nasopharyngeal carcinoma

73. A young adult presents to the emergency department after a motorcycle crash. The patient has bruises around the left orbital area and left temporal region. Examination notes alcoholic breath and GCS is 13 on arrival. Shortly afterwards, his GCS drops to 7. What is the single most important initial assessment?
    (A) MRI brain
    (B) CT head
    (C) CXR
    (D) Complete blood count
    (E) Blood grouping and matching

74. A child has just recovered from meningitis. What investigation will you do before discharge?
    (A) CT scan
    (B) EEG
    (C) Blood culture
    (D) Repeat lumber puncture
    (E) Hearing test

75. A 68 year old woman has a sudden onset of pain and loss of hearing in her left ear and unsteadiness when walking. There are small lesions visible on her palate and left external auditory meatus. What is the single most likely diagnosis?
    (A) Acute mastoiditis
    (B) Cholesteatoma
    (C) Herpes zoster infection
    (D) Oropharyngeal malignancy
    (E) Otitis media with effusion

76. A 26 year old woman has become aware of increasing right sided hearing impairment since her recent pregnancy. Her ear drums are normal. Hearing test shows bone conduction is better than air conduction. Weber's test lateralizes to the right ear. What is the single most likely diagnosis?
(A) Encephalopathy
(B) Functional hearing loss
(C) Tympanosclerosis
(D) Otosclerosis
(E) Sensorineural deafness

77. A 67 year old man with history of weight loss complaints of hoarseness of voice. CT reveals opacity in the right upper mediastinum. He denied any history of difficulty in breathing. What is the single most appropriate investigation?
(A) Laryngoscopy
(B) Bronchoscopy
(C) Lymph node biopsy
(D) Broncho alveolar lavage
(E) Barium swallow

78. A 10 year old girl has been referred for assessment of hearing as she is finding difficulty in hearing her teacher in the class. Her hearing test shows: bone conduction is normal, symmetrical air conduction threshold reduced bilaterally, Weber's test shows no lateralization. What is the single most likely diagnosis?
(A) Chronic perforation of tympanic membrane
(B) Chronic secretory otitis media with effusion
(C) Congenital sensorineural deficit
(D) Otosclerosis
(E) Presbyacusis

79. A 4 year old boy has earache and fever. He has taken paracetamol several times. Now it's noticed that he increases the TV volume. His preschool hearing test shows symmetric hearing loss of 40 db. What is the most likely diagnosis?

(A) Otitis media with effusion
(B) Otitis externa
(C) Cholesteatoma
(D) Chronic suppurative otitis media
(E) Tonsillitis

80. A 75 year old man has left sided earache and discomfort when he swallows. There is ulceration at the back of his tongue and he has a palpable non tender cervical mass. What is the single most likely diagnosis?
(A) Acute mastoiditis
(B) Dental abscess
(C) Herpes zoster infection
(D) Oropharyngeal malignancy
(E) Tonsillitis

81. A 42 year old man has been tired and sleepy for the last few weeks in the morning. His work has started getting affected as he feels sleepy in the meetings. His BMI is 36. What is the single most likely diagnosis?
(A) Idiopathic hypersomnia
(B) Narcolepsy
(C) Chest hyperventilation syndrome
(D) Obstructive sleep apnea syndrome
(E) REM-related sleep disorder

82. A 25 year old woman complains of dizziness, nausea, vomiting, visual disturbances and anxiety which keep coming from time to time. Most of the attacks are associated with sudden change in posture. What is the most likely diagnosis?
(A) Panic disorder
(B) Carotid sinus syncope
(C) Benign paroxysmal positional vertigo
(D) Vertebrobasilar insufficiency
(E) Postural hypotension

83. Patient had a fight following which he noticed bleeding, ringing and hearing loss from one ear. What is the investigation of choice?
    (A) CT
    (B) Skull X rays
    (C) Otoscopy
    (D) MRI vestibule
    (E) Coagulation study

84. A mother presents her 6 months old son who is vocalizing. She has noticed that he doesn't respond to loud noises. His motor milestones are normal. What is the best management strategy?
    (A) Arrange hearing test
    (B) Assess development milestones
    (C) Reassure
    (D) Refer to speech therapist
    (E) MRI brain

85. A 5 year old girl has had an upper respiratory tract infection for 3 days and has been treated with paracetamol by her mother. For the last 12 hour, she has been hot and irritable with severe pain in her right ear. What is the most likely diagnosis?
    (A) Herpes zoster infection
    (B) Impacted ear wax
    (C) Mumps
    (D) Otitis media
    (E) Perforation of ear drum

86. A 6 year old child presented with drooling of saliva and severe stridor. He is febrile and sick looking. X rays neck in extension shows a thumb sign. Choose the single most likely diagnosis.
    (A) Acute laryngotracheobronchitis
    (B) URTI
    (C) Diphtheria

(D) Tonsillitis
(E) Acute epiglottitis

87. A mother presents with her 3 year old son who has indistinct nasal speech. He snores at night and has restless sleep. He is tired by day times. What is the best management strategy?
(A) Arrange hearing test
(B) Assess development milestones
(C) Refer to ENT surgeon
(D) Refer to speech therapist
(E) MRI brain

88. A patient presents with hemoptysis 7 days after tonsillectomy. What is the next step?
(A) Packing
(B) Oral antibiotics and discharge
(C) Admit and IV antibiotics
(D) Return to OT and explore
(E) Ice cream and cold fluids

89. You are on duty doctor in the emergency department when a mother brings her 2 years old son with one hour history of noisy breathing. She states that although he had mild coryza over the last week, he was improving and so they had gone to a children's picnic with nursery friends. Another parent has found him coughing and spluttering, and ever since his breathing has remained noisy. Although he appears well in the ED, his current observation demonstrates a raised respiratory rate and SPO2 is 91% on air. What is the most likely diagnosis?
(A) Anaphylaxis
(B) Acute laryngotracheobronchitis
(C) Foreign body aspiration
(D) Epiglottitis
(E) URTI

90. A patient with sensorineural hearing loss and loss of corneal reflex on the left side. What is the most definitive investigation?
(A) CT (internal auditory meatus)
(B) Nuclear imaging of brain
(C) MRI (internal auditory meatus)
(D) Radio isotope scan
(E) Skull X rays

91. A 45 year old woman presents with rotational vertigo, nausea and vomiting, especially on moving her head. She also had a similar episode 2 years back. These episodes typically follow an event of runny nose, cold, cough and fever. What is the most probable diagnosis?
(A) Acoustic neuroma
(B) Meniere's disease
(C) Labyrinthitis
(D) BPPV
(E) Vestibular neuritis

92. A child playing with toys suddenly develops breathlessness and stridor. Which investigation will lead to the diagnosis?
(A) Laryngoscopy
(B) CXR
(C) Peak flow meter
(D) ABG
(E) FBC

93. A 2 year old child is brought by his mother. The mother had hearing impairment in her early childhood and is now concerned about the child. What investigation would you do?
(A) Audiometry
(B) Distraction testing
(C) Scratch test
(D) Tuning fork test
(E) Mastoid X rays

94. A 35 year old man presents with balance problems, headache, sensory neural hearing loss and loss of corneal reflex on the left side. What is the most definitive investigation?
(A) CT scan of internal auditory meatus
(B) Nuclear imagine of the brain
(C) MRI of the internal auditory meatus
(D) MRI brain
(E) Skull X rays

95. A 68 year old man has had increasing dysphagia for solid food for 3 months and has lost 5 Kg in weight. What single investigation is most likely to lead to a definitive diagnosis?
(A) Barium swallow
(B) CXR
(C) CT chest
(D) Endoscopy and biopsy
(E) Video- fluoroscopy

96. A child is not breathing and intubation is failed. At what anatomical site should incision be made?
(A) Cricoid cartilage
(B) First tracheal cartilage
(C) Hyoid bone
(D) Thyroid cartilage
(E) Linea alba

97. A 32 year old man has been to Thailand and returned back with cervical lymphadenopathy and fever. What is the most likely infection he is suffering from?
(A) HIV
(B) EBV
(C) Typhoid
(D) Measles
(E) Malaria

98. A 17 year old man has acute pain around his right eye, pain on one side of his face and earache too. What is the single most likely diagnosis?
(A) Ear wax
(B) Ear foreign body
(C) Dental abscess
(D) Cellulitis
(E) Herpes zoster

99. A 13 year old girl complains of a 2 day history of hoarseness of voice associated with cough. She feels feverish. On direct laryngoscopy, her vocal cords are grossly edematous. What is the single most appropriate next step?
(A) Conservative treatment
(B) Sputum for AFB
(C) Laryngoscopy
(D) Bronchoscopy
(E) Cervical spine X rays

100. A 6 year old child fell on his face 2 days ago. His parents have now brought him with difficulty in breathing. Examination shows fever, nasal bones are straight. What is the single most likely diagnosis?
(A) Nasal polyps
(B) Septal hematoma
(C) Septal abscess
(D) Deviated nasal septum
(E) Fracture nasal bone

101. A 4 year old child is brought to the emergency department by ambulance. His mother reports that he has been unwell with a sore throat for 8 hours. He is sitting on his mother's knee and is tolerating an oxygen mask but looks unwell. He has constant noisy breathing and he is drooling saliva. His temperature is 39C. What is the most important diagnosis?

(A) Acute asthma
(B) Bronchiolitis
(C) Acute laryngotracheobronchitis
(D) Epiglottitis
(E) Tonsillitis

102.   A middle age man who has had a history of chronic sinusitis, nasal obstruction and blood stained nasal discharge. He now presents with cheek swelling, epiphora, ptosis, diplopia and maxillary pain. What is the most likely diagnosis?
(A) Nasopharyngeal carcinoma
(B) Pharyngeal carcinoma
(C) Sinus squamous cell carcinoma
(D) Squamous cell laryngeal carcinoma
(E) Hypo pharyngeal tumor

103.   A 60 year old man with a long history of smoking and alcohol drinking presents with nasal obstruction, epistaxis, diplopia, otalgia and conductive deafness. What is the single most likely diagnosis?
(A) Nasopharyngeal carcinoma
(B) Pharyngeal carcinoma
(C) Sinus squamous cell carcinoma
(D) Squamous cell laryngeal carcinoma
(E) Hypo pharyngeal tumor

104.   A 34 year old man had a cold 2 days back. He now presents with right sided facial pain. What is the single most likely diagnosis?
(A) Maxillary sinusitis
(B) Ethmoid sinusitis
(C) Septal hematoma
(D) Septal abscess
(E) Allergic rhinitis

105.   A 29 year old man with a history of bronchial asthma comes with post nasal discharge and bilateral painless nasal blockage. What is the single most likely diagnosis?
(A) Nasal polyp
(B) Septal hematoma
(C) Septal abscess
(D) Atopic rhinitis
(E) Allergic rhinitis

106.   A 64 year old man presents with ipsilateral vertigo, tinnitus and left sided hearing loss. On exam; Rinne's test is positive and Weber's test lateralizes to the right ear. What is the most appropriate investigation?
(A) CT
(B) MRI brain
(C) Mastoid X rays
(D) Audiometry
(E) Caloric test

107.   A young man was knocked down during a fight in the waiting room of the emergency department. He is now unconscious and unresponsive. What is the first thing you would do?
(A) Set up IV line
(B) Put oropharyngeal airway
(C) Endotracheal intubation
(D) Assess GCS
(E) Start CPR

108.   A man had a soft mass on his mandible. Mass is freely mobile and has started growing progressively over the past 6 months. The mass still moves freely. What is the best investigation for this patient?
(A) FNAC
(B) CT
(C) X rays
(D) MRI

(E) ESR

109.   A 4 year old boy presents with fever, severe ear ache, vomiting and anorexia. He also has tonsillitis. On examination, tympanic membranes are bulging. He came to the GP a few days ago and was diagnosed with URTI. What is the single most appropriate diagnosis?
(A) Otitis externa
(B) Acute otitis media
(C) Serous otitis media
(D) Chronic suppurative otitis media
(E) Mastoiditis

110.   A 67 year old builder presents with a persistent nodular lesion on upper part of pinna with some telangiectasia around the lesion. What is the most possible diagnosis?
(A) Basal cell carcinoma
(B) Squamous cell carcinoma
(C) Keratoacanthoma
(D) Actinic keratosis
(E) Melanoma

111.   A young child was brought by his mother to the OPD complaining that he raised the volume of the television and didn't response to her when she called him. On examination, tympanic membrane was dull greyish and no shadow of handle of malleus. What is the most probable diagnosis?
(A) Chronic otitis media
(B) Acute otitis media
(C) Secretory otitis media
(D) Otitis externa
(E) Cholesteatoma

112.   A 73 tear old man who was a chronic smoker has quit smoking for the past 3 years ago. He now presents with hoarseness of voice and cough since past 3 weeks. On chest

X rays, mass is visible in the mediastinum. What is the best investigation to confirm the diagnosis?
(A) Bronchoscopy
(B) Thoracoscopy
(C) Ultrasound
(D) CT thorax
(E) Lymph node biopsy

113.   A 25 year old woman has recent cough, hoarseness and swelling in the neck. There are several non-tender swellings on both sides of her neck. She has lost 13 Kg. She takes recreational drugs. What is the most probable diagnosis?
(A) Thyrotoxicosis
(B) Hyperthyroidism
(C) Vocal cord nodules
(D) Carcinoma bronchus
(E) Tuberculosis

114.   A 35 year old man presents with a headache that worsens on bending his head forward. What is the most likely diagnosis?
(A) Chronic sinusitis
(B) Subarachnoid hemorrhage
(C) Migraine
(D) Cluster headache
(E) Tension headache

115.   A 20 year old man presents with painful swallowing. On examination, he has trismus and unilateral enlargement of his tonsils. The Peritonsillar region is red, inflamed and swollen. What is the most appropriate treatment?
(A) Oral antibiotics
(B) IV antibiotics and analgesics
(C) I&D with antibiotics
(D) Analgesics with antipyretics
(E) Tonsillectomy

116.   A 20 year old woman with no previous history of ear problem presents with one day history of severe pain in the right ear which is extremely tender to examine. What is the single most likely diagnosis?
(A) Chondromalacia
(B) Furunculosis
(C) Myringitis
(D) Otitis externa
(E) Otitis media

117.   A 36 year old woman has an injury to the right external laryngeal nerve during a thyroid surgery. What symptom would be expected in this patient?
(A) Stridor
(B) Hoarseness
(C) Aphonia
(D) Dysphonia
(E) Aphasia

118.   A 75 year old woman has weakness of the left side of her face. She has had a painful ear for 48 hours. There are pustules in the left ear canal and on the ear drum. What is the single most likely diagnosis?
(A) Chronic serous otitis media
(B) Herpes zoster infection
(C) Impacted ear wax
(D) Perforation of ear drum
(E) Presbyacusis

119.   A 45 year old woman has dull aching pain in her right ear which has been presented for a several weeks. There is no discharge from the effected ear. Chewing is uncomfortable and her husband has noticed that she grinds her teeth during sleep. The ear drum appears normal. What is the single most likely diagnosis?
(A) Dental caries

(B) Mumps
(C) Otitis media
(D) Temporomandibular joint pain
(E) Trigeminal neuralgia

120.   A child distressed with fever, stridor and unable to swallow saliva. His respiratory rate is 40 beats per minutes. What is the initial step that needs to be taken?
(A) Examine throat
(B) Secure airway
(C) Keep him laid flat
(D) IV penicillin
(E) IV fluids

ANSWER KEYS

1	A	11	B	21	D	31	A	41	D	51	E
2	D	12	E	22	D	32	B	42	B	52	B
3	B	13	A	23	C	33	D	43	C	53	A
4	D	14	D	24	B	34	E	44	C	54	D
5	A	15	C	25	D	35	E	45	B	55	B
6	A	16	C	26	A	36	D	46	B	56	C
7	E	17	D	27	D	37	B	47	D	57	C
8	B	18	A	28	B	38	D	48	B	58	D
9	C	19	D	29	D	39	B	49	A	59	A
10	D	20	A	30	C	40	D	50	C	60	B

61	B	71	C	81	D	91	E	101	D	111	C
62	C	72	A	82	C	92	A	102	C	112	E
63	A	73	B	83	C	93	A	103	A	113	E
64	E	74	E	84	A	94	D	104	A	114	A
65	C	75	C	85	D	95	D	105	A	115	C
66	E	76	D	86	E	96	A	106	B	116	D
67	D	77	C	87	C	97	B	107	B	117	D
68	E	78	B	88	C	98	E	108	A	118	B
69	B	79	A	89	C	99	A	109	C	119	D
70	C	80	D	90	C	100	C	110	A	120	B

1. **The causative agent in otomycosis is:**
   a. Aspergillus niger & / or Candida albicans.
   b. Streptococci.
   c. Staphylococci
   d. E.coli
   e. B. pyocyaneus.

2. **Bloody discharge from the ear occurs in:**
   a. Fracture base of the skull.
   b. Glomus jugular tumor.
   c. Haemorrhagic otitis media.
   d. Rupture drum.
   e. All of the above.

3. **In traumatic ossicular disruption, all is true EXCEPT:**
   a. The audiogram shows 55 dB loss.
   b. Separation of the incudo-stapedial joint is the commonest lesion.
   c. There is bulging drum.
   d. C.T scan is indicated.
   e. The audiogram shows no sensorineural hearing loss.

4. **Gradenigo syndrome occurs in:**
   a. Acute mastoid abscess.
   b. Acute petrositis.
   c. Chronic otitis media.
   d. Secretory otitis media.
   e. Fracture base of the skull.

5. **Tobey-Ayer's test is a characteristic sign in:**
   a. Brain abscess.
   b. Lateral sinus thrombosis.
   c. Extradural abscess.
   d. Meningitis.
   e. Cavernous sinus thrombosis.

6. **Pain in acute tonsillitis is referred to the ear through:**
   a. The 5th nerve.
   b. The 9th nerve.
   c. The 10th nerve.
   d. The 7th nerve.
   e. The 2nd & 3rd cervical nerve.

7. **The fluids presents in secretory otitis media is:**
   a. Mucopurulent.
   b. Serosanguinous.
   c. Exudates.
   d. Transudates.
   e. Mixture of exudates & transudates.

8. **In Weber's test:**
   a. In conductive deafness: sound is heard better in the diseased ear.
   b. In conductive deafness: sound is heard better in the healthy ear.
   c. In bilateral conductive deafness: sound is heard better in the better hearing ear.
   d. In perceptive deafness: sound is heard worse in the healthy ear.
   e. In perceptive deafness: sound is heard better in the diseased ear.

9. **The following is true about impedance audiometry EXCEPT:**
   a. It measures the pressure changes in the middle ear.
   b. It measures the fixation of the ossicular chain.
   c. It measures the dislocation of the ossicular chain.
   d. It measures the patency of the Eustachian tube.
   e. It measures the sound emitted from the cochlea.

10. **In lesion of the facial nerve at horizontal part, there will be the following problem EXCEPT:**
    a. Loss of taste.
    b. Impairment of salivation.
    c. Impairment of lacrimation.
    d. Loss of stapedial reflex.
    e. Impairment of wrinkling of forehead.

11. **The early symptom of Bell's palsy is:**
    a. Dropping of angle of the affected side.
    b. Difficulty in eye closure.
    c. Obliteration of the angle of the mouth.
    d. Pain of acute onset behind the ear.
    e. Loss of stapedial reflex.

12. **In malignant otitis externa all the following is true EXCEPT:**
    a. It is common in old diabetic.
    b. There may be facial paralysis.
    c. The commonest organism is pseudomonas.
    d. Mainly treated surgically.
    e. Ciprofloxacin is the drug of choice.
13. **Longitudinal fracture of the temporal bone may be associated with all of the following EXCEPT:**
    a. LMNL facial palsy.
    b. Traumatic perforation of the tympanic membrane.
    c. Conductive hearing loss.
    d. Profound hearing loss.
    e. Ossicular injury including incudostapedal dislocation.
14. **ABR "Auditory Brain stem Response" is used in:**
    a. Infants as a screening test.
    b. Test of hearing in malingering.
    c. Test of hearing in retrocochlear lesion.
    d. Detection of acoustic neuroma.
    e. All of the above.
15. **In traumatic rupture of the drum, all are true EXCEPT:**
    a. The main treatment is conservative.
    b. Local ear drops are highly indicated.
    c. It heals spontaneously within 3 months.
    d. It may be caused by longitudinal fracture of the temporal bone.
    e. Topical antibiotic is contraindicated.
16. **Early acute suppurative otitis media is manifested by:**
    a. Retracted tympanic membrane.
    b. Aural fullness.
    c. Deafness.
    d. Earache.
    e. All of the above.
17. **The most accurate diagnostic test to detect degeneration of the facial nerve:**
    a. Nerve excitability test.
    b. Electromyography.

    c. Electroneurography.

    d. Stapedial reflex.

    e. Ultrasonography.

18. **Unilateral hearing loss with pulsating tinnitus is suggestive of:**

    a. Otosclerosis.

    b. Extradural abscess complicating CSOM.

    c. Glomus tumor.

    d. Acoustic neuroma.

    e. Carotid body tumour.

19. **The most common cause of vertigo is:**

    a. Acoustic neuroma.

    b. Ototoxicity.

    c. Meniere's disease.

    d. Benign paroxysmal positional vertigo.

    e. Vestibular neuronitis.

20. **A case of ear infection followed by headache, blurring of vision & vomiting is suggestive of:**

    a. Mastoiditis.

    b. Petrositis.

    c. Labyrinthitis.

    d. Brain abscess.

    e. Lateral sinus thrombophlebitis.

21. **Mixed hearing loss may be caused by one of the following:**

    a. Otosclerosis.

    b. Meniere's disease.

    c. Ear wax.

    d. Acoustic neuroma.

    e. Ossicular disruption.

22. **Pulsating ear discharge may be found in:**

    a. Extradural abscess.

    b. Acute exacerbation of CSOM.

    c. Acute otitis media with small perforation.

    d. Acute mastoiditis with tympanic membrane perforation.

    e. All of the above.

23. **The triad of ear discharge, retro-orbital pain and 6th nerve paralysis is due to:**
    a. Mastoiditis.
    b. Labyrinthitis.
    c. Apical petrositis.
    d. Lateral sinus thrombosis.
    e. Longitudinal fracture of temporal bone.
24. **In case of Meniere's disease with mild SNHL is treated by all the following EXCEPT:**
    a. Medical treatment.
    b. Labyrinthectomy.
    c. Endolymphatic sac decompression.
    d. Vestibular nerve section.
    e. Lifestyle modification.
25. **Nystagmus & vertigo induced by pressure on the tragus is a sign of:**
    a. Fistula complicating cholesteatoma.
    b. Benign paroxysmal vertigo.
    c. Vestibular neuritis.
    d. Cholesteatoma only.
    e. Perilymph fistula.
26. **Insertion of Grommet tube is indicated in:**
    a. Acute suppurative otitis media.
    b. Secretory otitis media resistant to medical treatment.
    c. Chronic otitis media.
    d. Acute mastoiditis.
    e. Barotraumatic otitis media.
27. **Acute mastoiditis is manifested by all of the following EXCEPT:**
    a. Tenderness over mastoid antrum.
    b. Continuous ear discharge.
    c. Sagging of postero-superior meatal wall.
    d. Obliteration of retro-auricular sulcus.
    e. Mastoid erythema.
28. **Vertigo in a case of cholesteatoma is suggestive of:**
    a. Temporal lobe abscess.
    b. Acute petrositis.

c. Lateral sinus thrombosis.

d. Labyrinthine fistula.

e. Facial nerve palsy.

29. **Equilibrium during angular "rotational" movement is the function of:**

    a. The utricle.

    b. The saccule.

    c. The cochlea.

    d. The semicircular canal.

    e. Cerebellum.

30. **Facial palsy is most commonly:**

    a. Neoplastic.

    b. Traumatic.

    c. Herpetic.

    d. Bell's palsy.

    e. With cholesteatoma.

31. **A false +ve fistula test is due to:**

    a. Labyrinthine fistula with dead ear.

    b. Cholesteatoma bridging an inner ear fistula.

    c. Hyper mobile footplate of the stapes.

    d. Perilymph fistula.

    e. All of the above.

32. **The concept that the facial nerve supplies the auricle is related to:**

    a. Ramsey-Hunt syndrome.

    b. Jugular foramen syndrome.

    c. Horner's syndrome.

    d. Bell's palsy.

    e. Coughing with ear cleaning.

33. **The most common cause of otitis media with effusion is:**

    a. Inadequate treatment of acute otitis media.

    b. Nasopharyngeal neoplasm.

    c. Allergy.

    d. Otitic barotrauma.

    e. Cleft palate.

34. **A patient with uncomplicated CSOM has:**

    a. Ear discharge & headache.

b. Ear discharge & dizziness.

c. Ear discharge & hearing impairment.

d. Ear discharge & fever.

e. Hearing impairment & dizziness.

35. Mikulicz cell is a characteristic histological finding in:

a. Rhinoscleroma.

b. Rhinosporidiosis.

c. Aspergillosis.

d. Sarcoidosis.

e. Mikulicz disease.

36. Russell bodies is a characteristic histological finding in:

a. Rhinoscleroma.

b. Rhinosporidiosis.

c. Aspergillosis.

d. Sarcoidosis.

e. Mucormycosis.

37. Perforation of bony part of the nasal septum occurs in:

a. Sarcoidosis.

b. Rhinoscleroma.

c. Tuberculosis.

d. Syphilis.

e. Septal abscess.

38. The causative agent of rhinoscleroma is:

a. Sporozoon.

b. Low virulent TB bacillus.

c. Treponema pallidum.

d. Gram negative short capsulated diplobacillus.

e. Chlamydia.

39. The causative agent of lupus vulgaris is:

a. Sporozoon.

b. Low virulent T.B bacillus.

c. Treponema pallidum.

d. Gram negative short capsulated diplobacillus.

e. Mycoplasma.

40. F.B of nose is represented by:

a. Bilateral nasal obstruction.

b. Unilateral nasal discharge.

c. Bilateral nasal epistaxis.

d. Unilateral nasal obstruction and discharge.

e. Recurrent epistaxis.

41. The mechanism of nasal allergy is:

    a. Type 1 hypersensitivity reaction.

    b. Type 2 hypersensitivity reaction.

    c. Type 3 hypersensitivity reaction.

    d. Type 4 hypersensitivity reaction.

    e. Combination of type 1 and type 3 hypersensitivity reaction.

42. The most common type of nasal polypi is:

    a. Allergic.

    b.   Infective.

    c. Secondary to malignancy in the nose.

    d. Cystic fibrosis.

    e. Kartagener syndrome.

43. All the following lines of treatment could be applied in rhinoscleroma EXCEPT:

    a. Rifampicin.

    b. Cytotoxic drugs.

    c. Surgery to canalize the stenosed canal.

    d. Laser surgery.

44. Unilateral polypoidal mass arising from the lateral wall of the nose in 55 years old man is most probably:

    a. Inverted papilloma.

    b. Rhinoscleroma.

    c. Allergic nasal polyp.

    d. Antrochoanal polyp.

    e. Rhinophyma.

45. The most common site of origin of allergic nasal polypi is:

    a. Maxillary sinus.

    b. Ethmoidal sinus.

    c. Frontal sinus.

    d. Sphenoid sinus.

    e. Ethmoidal bulla.

46. CSF rhinorrhea is characterized by all of the following EXCEPT:

a. Clear color.
b. Sediment formation after standing in a test tube.
c. Containing glucose.
d. Accelerated flow rate with straining.
e. Containing beta-2 transferrin.

47. **Perforation of the cartilaginous part of the nasal septum may be due to:**
    a. Rhinoscleroma.
    b. Sarcoidosis.
    c. T.B.
    d. Syphilis.
    e. Rhinolith.

48. **Radiological finding of sinusitis include all of the following EXCEPT:**
    a. Bone destruction.
    b. Opacity of the affected sinus.
    c. Fluid level.
    d. Mucosal thickening.

49. **The main presenting symptom of ethmoidal nasal polyp are all of the following EXCEPT:**
    a. Attack of severe epistaxis.
    b. Persistent nasal obstruction.
    c. Rhinorrhea.
    d. Facial pain or headache
    e.   Hyposmia.

50. **Which of the following is used to confirm nasal allergy:**
    a. Eosinophilia in nasal secretion.
    b. Eosinophilia in blood.
    c. Elevated serum IgE.
    d. All of the above.

51. **Nasal regurgitation occurs in all of the following EXCEPT:**
    a. Ethmoid carcinoma.
    b. Palatal paralysis.
    c. Advanced maxillary sinus carcinoma.
    d. Cleft palate.

e. Post-operatively after nasopharyngeal angiofibroma operation.

52. **Unilateral nasal obstruction in newly born infant may be due to:**
    a. Antrochoanal polyp.
    b. Allergic nasal polyp.
    c. Choanal atresia.
    d. Foreign body in the nose.
    e. Laryngeal stenosis.

53. **Unilateral mucopurulent nasal discharge in a child may be due to:**
    a. Unilateral sinusitis.
    b. FB in the nose.
    c. Antrochoanal polyp.
    d. Allergic rhinitis.
    e. Cystic fibrosis.

54. **The frontal mucocele may be caused by:**
    a. Chronic frontal sinusitis.
    b. Obstruction of a duct of a mucus gland.
    c. Obstruction of frontal sinus ostium.
    d. Frontal osteoma.
    e. All of the above.

55. **The following are some general causes of epistaxis EXCEPT:**
    a. Anaemia.
    b. Arterial hypertension.
    c. Nasopharyngeal angiofibroma.
    d. Renal failure.
    e. Chronic liver disease.

56. **The most common site of nasal bleeding is:**
    a. Little's area.
    b. MacEwen triangle.
    c. Pyriform fossa.
    d. Sphenoethmoidal recess.
    e. Woodruff's Plexus.

57. **Resistant epistaxis from below the middle turbinate requires ligation of:**

a. The anterior ethmoidal artery.
b. The sphenopalatine artery.
c. The posterior ethmoidal artery.
d. The maxillary artery.
e. The external carotid artery.

58. **Nasopharyngeal carcinoma cause Horner's syndrome as a result of infiltration of:**
    a. The 3rd cranial nerve.
    b. The 5th cranial nerve.
    c. The 7th cranial nerve.
    d. The 9th cranial nerve.
    e. Cervical sympathetic chain.

59. **The following drugs can cause epistaxis EXCEPT:**
    a. Salicylates.
    b. Anticoagulants.
    c. Quinine.
    d. Ampicillin.
    e. Cocaine.

60. **The following lesions may leads to proptosis EXCEPT:**
    a. Nasopharyngeal angiofibroma.
    b. Nasopharyngeal carcinoma.
    c. Adenoid hypertrophy.
    d. Nasopharyngeal sarcoma.
    e. Frontal mucocele.

61. **The commonest cause of CSF rhinorrhea is:**
    a. Congenital.
    b. Traumatic.
    c. Infective.
    d. Neoplastic.
    e. Idiopathic.

62. **Cyclic asphyxia is the presenting symptom is:**
    a. Bilateral choanal atresia.
    b. Adenoids.
    c. Acute laryngitis.
    d. Nasal allergy.
    e. Laryngomalacia.

63. **The commonest cause of epistaxis in 50 years old man is:**

a. Hypertension.
b. Angiofibroma.
c. Trauma.
d. Rhinosinusitis.
e. Inverted papilloma.

64. The point of tenderness in acute frontal sinusitis is:
a. The inner canthus.
b. The outer canthus.
c. The supra-orbital margin.
d. The infra-orbital margin.
e. The floor of the frontal sinus immediately above the inner canthus.

65. The point of tenderness in acute ethmoidal sinusitis is:
a. The inner canthus.
b. The outer canthus.
c. The supra-orbital margin.
d. The infra-orbital margin.
e. None of them.

66. Unilateral nasal discharge and unilateral nasal obstruction in 13 years old boy is most probably diagnostic of:
a. Choanal atresia.
b. Adenoids.
c. Nasopharyngeal carcinoma.
d. Antrochoanal polyp.
e. Nasopharyngeal angiofibroma.

67. Watery fluid in the maxillary sinus indicates:
a. Suppurative inflammation with irreversible mucosal damage.
b. Suppurative inflammation with reversible pathology.
c. Allergic sinusitis.
d. Catarrhal inflammation.
e. Cystic fibrosis.

68. In a case of 5 years old boy with a membranous faucial lesion, temp 38° & pulse 180/min, the most probable diagnosis is:
a. Infectious mononucleosis.

b. Acute follicular tonsillitis.
c. Faucial diphtheria.
d. Agranulocytosis.
e. Candidal infection of tonsils.

69. **Membranous tonsillitis may be due to:**
    a. Faucial diphtheria.
    b. Candidal infection of tonsils.
    c. Acute follicular tonsillitis.
    d. Infectious mononucleosis.
    e. All of the above.

70. **The following antibiotic is contraindicated in infectious mononucleosis:**
    a. Ampicillin.
    b. Erythromycin.
    c. Cephalosporin.
    d. Ciprofloxacin.
    e. Amoxicillin.

71. **Adenoid hypertrophy may lead to all of the following EXCEPT:**
    a. Adenoid facies.
    b. Otitis media with effusion.
    c. Sensory neural deafness.
    d. Night mares.

72. **Chronic retropharyngeal abscess is treated by:**
    a. External drainage posterior to sternomastoid.
    b. External drainage anterior to sternomastoid.
    c. Internal drainage via longitudinal incision.
    d. None of the above.

73. **Acute retropharyngeal abscess is treated by:**
    a. External drainage posterior to sternomastoid.
    b. External drainage anterior to sternomastoid.
    c. Internal drainage via longitudinal incision.
    d. None of the above.

74. **Juvenile nasopharyngeal angiofibroma spread to the surrounding tissue because it is:**
    a. Malignant.
    b. Non capsulated.

c. Pre-malignant.

d. Highly vascular.

75. Juvenile nasopharyngeal angiofibroma may cause:

    a. Conductive deafness.

    b. Sensory neural deafness.

    c. Mixed deafness.

    d. All of the above.

76. The most dangerous complication of Ludwig`s angina is:

    a. Acute laryngeal edema.

    b. CHL.

    c. Bleeding.

    d. Nasal obstruction.

77. Trotter's syndrome occurs in:

    a. Nasopharyngeal carcinoma.

    b. Oropharyngeal carcinoma.

    c. Hypopharyngeal carcinoma.

    d. Postcricoid carcinoma.

78. Sixth cranial nerve paralysis occurs in the following cases EXCEPT:

    a. Nasopharyngeal carcinoma.

    b. Cavernous sinus thrombosis.

    c. Postcricoid carcinoma.

    d. Petrositis.

79. Pain in the ear in cases of acute tonsillitis or following tonsillectomy is referred via:

    a. The 5th nerve.

    b. The 9th nerve.

    c. The 10th nerve.

    d. The 12th nerve.

80. The cause of reactionary hemorrhage after tonsillectomy:

    a. Secondary infection.

    b. Rising blood pressure with slipping of ligature.

    c. Injury of the pharyngeal muscles & mucosa.

    d. None of the above.

81. Infection reaching the submental & submandibular space is called:

    a. Vincent angina.

b. Ludwig's angina.

c. Submandibular sialadenitis.

d. Bezold's abscess.

82. **Behcet's disease is characterized by all of the following EXCEPT:**

   a. Stomatitis, herpes like lesion.

   b. Conjunctivitis, corneal opacity, iridocyclitis.

   c. Genital ulcer.

   d. SNHL.

   e. Tendency to recur.

83. **Bull neck is known to occur in:**

   a. Tonsillar diphtheria.

   b. Quinsy.

   c. Acute tonsillitis.

   d. Chronic tonsillitis.

84. **The dysphagia in Plummer-Vinson syndrome start to:**

   a. Solids then to fluids.

   b. Fluids then to solids.

   c. Fluid & solids at the same time.

   d. All of the above.

85. **The dysphagia in cardiac achalasia starts to:**

   a. Solids then to fluids.

   b. Fluids then to solids.

   c. Fluid & solids at the same time.

   d. All of the above.

86. **The anemia in Plummer Vinson syndrome is:**

   a. Microcytic hypochromic.

   b. Macrocytic normochromic.

   c. Macrocytic hypochromic.

   d. Normocytic normochromic.

87. **Dysphagia lusoria is:**

   a. Compression of the oesophagus by abnormally located RT subclavian artery or double aorta.

   b. Herniation of the pharyngeal mucosa via Killian dehiscence.

   c. Chronic superficial oesophagitis with web formation.

   d. Failure of relaxation of cardiac sphincter.

88. **The cause of death in corrosive oesophagitis may be:**
    a. Dehydration due to electrolytes imbalance.
    b. Stridor due to laryngeal oedema.
    c. Oesophageal perforation.
    d. Hypovolaemic shock.

89. **Pharyngeal pouch occurs mostly in:**
    a. Old males.
    b. Old females.
    c. Infants.
    d. Adult males.

90. **Violent vomiting or large meal may cause:**
    a. Pharyngeal pouch.
    b. Cardiac achalasia.
    c. Spontaneous rupture of the oesophagus.
    d. Plummer Vinson syndrome.

91. **Apnoea immediately after opening the trachea is due to:**
    a. Rise of the blood carbon dioxide level.
    b. Rise of the blood O_2 level.
    c. Wash of the blood carbon dioxide level.
    d. Fall of the blood O_2 level.

92. **Inhaled smooth small FB is commonly arrested in:**
    a. The larynx.
    b. The trachea.
    c. The right main bronchus.
    d. The left main bronchus.

93. **30 years old female suffering from bilateral nasal obstruction, crusty nose, hoarseness of voice & stridor. The most probable cause is:**
    a. Allergic rhinitis.
    b. Vasomotor rhinitis.
    c. Rhinolaryngoscleroma.
    d. Acute rhinosinusitis.

94. **The commonest cause of breathing difficulty after tracheostomy is:**
    a. Pneumonia.
    b. Obstruction of the tube by secretion.
    c. Surgical emphysema.

    d. Pneumothorax.

95. The causative agent of acute laryngotracheobronchitis is:
    a. Pneumococci.
    b. Staphylococci.
    c. Streptococcus haemolyticus.
    d. Human parainfluenza viruses.

96. The following conditions cause stridor EXCEPT:
    a. Laryngeal diphtheria.
    b. Acute laryngitis in adult.
    c. Acute laryngitis in children.
    d. Multiple laryngeal papilloma.

97. Mediastinal emphysema after tracheostomy occurs due to:
    a. When the pretracheal fascia is sutured tightly.
    b. Injury of the pleura.
    c. A small tracheal tear.
    d. Cricoid cartilage damage.

98. Dyspnea, crepitation and expectoration of large amount of frothy stained sputum after tracheostomy is suspected of:
    a. Pneumothorax.
    b. Acute pulmonary edema.
    c. Mediastinal emphysema.
    d. Tracheobronchial fistula.

99. Ulceration of the vocal cord edge (mouse nibbled) occurs in:
    a. Tuberculosis.
    b. Scleroma.
    c. Syphilis.
    d. Sarcoidosis.

100.   Laryngeal stenosis may be due to:
    a. Perichondritis.
    b. Endotracheal intubation.
    c. Syphilis.
    d. All of the above.

101.   The most common parotid lesion in children is:
    a. mixed tumor

b. lymphangioma and hemangioma
c. lymphoma
d. mucoepidermoid carcinoma
e. Warthin's tumor.

102. **Warthin's tumor of the parotid is most common in:**
   a. The tail of the parotid in females over 60 years old.
   b. The tail of the parotid in males over 60 years old.
   c. The superficial lobe, equally distributed in both sexes.
   d. The deep lobe in females.
   e. Young adult males.

103. **Pleomorphic adenoma of the salivary glands consists of:**
   a. Ductal elements only.
   b. Predominance of lymphocytes.
   c. Epithelial and myoepithelial elements.
   d. Cartilage rest cells.
   e. None of the above.

104. **A patient of phonasthenia shows elliptical space between vocal cords on indirect laryngoscopy; which of the following muscle is involved?**
   a. Interarytenoid.
   b. Thyroarytenoid.
   c. Cricothyroid.
   d. Thyroepiglottic.

105. **In a patient presenting to the emergency room with fractured nose associated with edema:**
   a. Postpone reduction for one week.
   b. Immediate reduction of the nasal fracture is needed.
   c. Patient should be prepared for immediate septorhinoplasty.
   d. Postpone for one month before reduction.

106. **Oroantral fistula may follow all of the following EXCEPT:**
   a. Extraction of upper 2nd premolar tooth.
   b. Radical antrostomy operation.
   c. Advanced maxillary carcinoma.
   d. Inferior meatal antrostomy.

107.   A patient presented with bilateral nasal obstruction after nasal trauma. The patient temperature is 38. There is throbbing nasal pain. Your diagnosis is:
   a. Nasal furunculosis.
   b. Septal hematoma.
   c. Septal abscess.
   d. Septal perforation.

108.   A 40-year-old male presented with left nasal obstruction and fleshy reddish nasal mass. There is a history of recurrence after previous surgery 2 years ago. The likely diagnosis is:
   a. Nasopharyngeal angiofibroma
   b. Inverted papilloma.
   c. Allergic nasal polyps.
   d. Bleeding polypus of nasal septum.

109.   A 3-year-old male child with recurrent epistaxis, subcutaneous hematoma and swollen joints after minor trauma is probably suffering from:
   a. Thrombocytopenic purpura.
   b. Hemophilia.
   c. Leukemia.
   d. Rheumatic fever

Answer Key:

1. A	40. d	79. b
2. c	41. a	80. b
3. c	42. a	81. b
4. b	43. b	82. d
5. b	44. a	83. a
6. b	45. b	84. a
7. e	46. b	85. b
8. a	47. c	86. a
9. e	48. a	87. a
10. c	49. a	88. b
11. c	50. d	89. a
12. d	51. a	90. c
13. d	52. c	91. c
14. e	53. b	92. c
15. b	54. e	93. c
16. e	55. c	94. b
17. c	56. a	95. d
18. c	57. b	96. b
19. d	58. e	97. c
20. d	59. d	98. b
21. a	60. c	99. a
22. a	61. b	100. d
23. c	62. a	101. b
24. b	63. a	102. b
25. a	64. e	103. c
26. b	65. a	104. b
27. d	66. d	105. a
28. d	67. c	106. d
29. d	68. b	107. c
30. d	69. e	108. b
31. c	70. a	109. b
32. a	71. c	
33. a	72. a	
34. c	73. c	
35. a	74. b	
36. a	75. a	
37. d	76. a	
38. d	77. a	
39. b	78. c	

www.ingramcontent.com/pod-product-compliance
Lightning Source LLC
Chambersburg PA
CBHW071243220526
45468CB00002B/981